Modern Tai Chi

Tobias Block

MODERN TAI CHI

Only 15 minutes to your healthy life!

1st edition

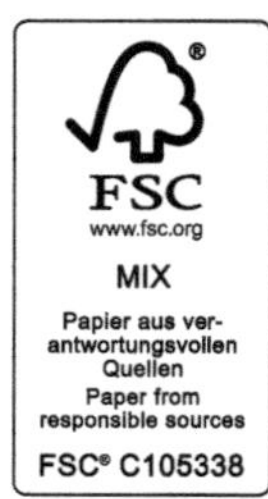

Bibliographic information of the German National Library:
The German National Library lists this publication in the German National Bibliography; detailed bibliographic data can be accessed on the Internet at http://dnb.dnb.de.

Editorial office: Dr rer. nat. Henning Schweer

Publisher: BoD · Books on Demand GmbH, In de Tarpen 42, 22848 Norderstedt
Print: Libri Plureos GmbH, Friedensallee 273, 22763 Hamburg

ISBN: 978-3-7597-7547-4

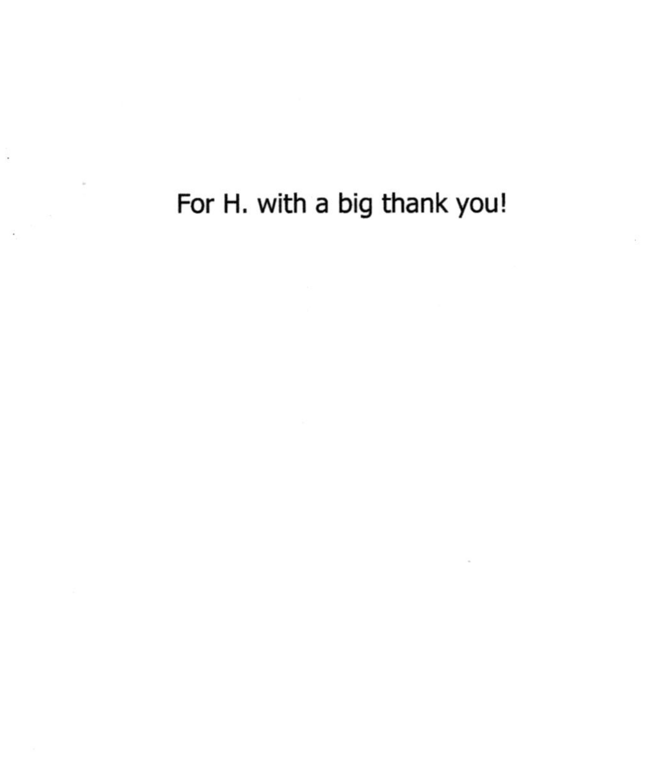

For H. with a big thank you!

Contents

Foreword

I can say without a doubt that this book and the Modern Tai Chi method presented in it will be of benefit to anyone in search of physical and mental relaxation and health. The programme presented by Tobias Block builds a bridge between the centuries-old tradition of Asia and our Western culture. For almost twenty years, countless people have learnt these simple yet highly effective exercises in Tobias Block's courses and have been using them in their everyday lives ever since.

I myself can confirm from years of practice that the full range of positive effects on muscles, breathing, concentration and mind can be experienced with just 15 minutes of daily practice. In contrast to many other methods of physical and mental exercise, Modern Tai Chi is very easy to integrate into everyday life. A quiet place and a few minutes of time, that's all it takes, no equipment, no mats, no gymnastics on the floor. Whether young or old, couch potato or sports ace, anyone and everyone can find an introduction to more peace and fitness with Modern Tai Chi.

I am delighted that Tobias Block has decided to present his concept of Modern Tai Chi to a wider audience with this book. With his many years of experience as a sports physician and personal trainer, he shows us Europeans a way to make the ancient health teachings of Tai Chi fruitful in our modern everyday lives.

I wish all readers every success on their journey to better health and well-being!

Dr rer. nat. Henning Schweer

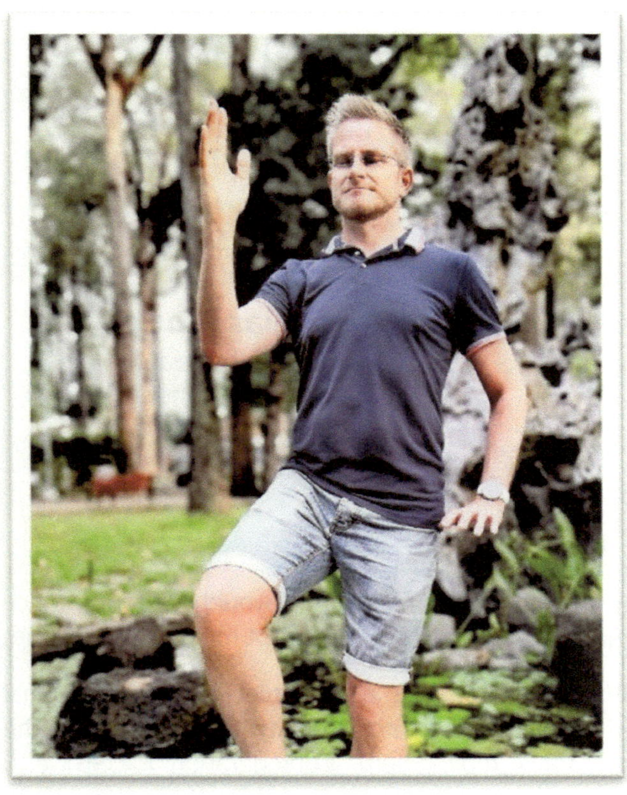

Modern Tai Chi:
Your path to better physical and mental health

1. Welcome to Modern Tai Chi

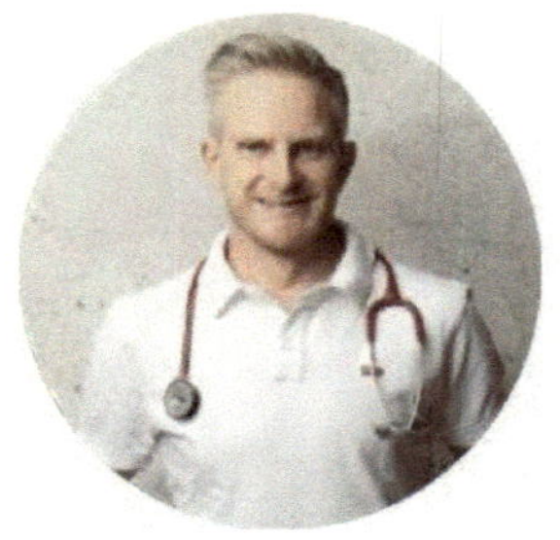

Tobias Block
sports physician,
personal trainer & lecturer

My name is Tobias Block and I would like to introduce you to my Modern Tai Chi concept for your healthy life.

After my active career as an athlete up to the national swimming squad, I completed my trainer training at the German Olympic Sports Confederation (DOSB) e.V. with the highest level - an A licence. At the same time, I laid the foundations for my current work by studying human medicine at the Christian-Albrechts-University (CAU) in Kiel and then journalism and moderation at the Hanseatic Academy for Marketing and Media (HAMM) in Hamburg. As a sports physician, personal trainer and lecturer, I work with people who want to improve their lives through movement!

I mainly work with private individuals, companies, studios and medical facilities in Germany and Sweden. This can be done live, on site or online in individual meetings or 24/7 via my video workouts.

You have been able to find me regularly offering my services on board the *Mein Schiff®* **fleet** since 2011. Since 2018, I have also been accompanying, supporting and motivating you on board the **Hapag-Lloyd Cruises fleet** with themed trips on 'Sport & Health'.

You can always find up-to-date information about me and my services at **www.fitcare.training** - or contact me at any time by email, WhatsApp or give me a call.

I wish you much joy in developing your Modern Tai Chi,

Tobias Block

2. Tai Chi comes from Asia

Tai Chi is a form of movement that originated in Asia. It originated centuries ago, has continued to develop ever since and is now spreading across the globe. More and more people are also trying out Tai Chi here in Europe. However, this often leads to disappointment and problems when learning and practising. The historically developed pictorial instructions of Asian learning are not familiar to us Europeans and are sometimes difficult to understand. As a result, beginners have no sense of achievement and stop training. This is where my concept of Modern Tai Chi comes in and helps us Europeans.

I break down Asian instructions such as 'move like a tree in the wind' into individual, structured and logical instructions. We can all manage instructions such as 'spread your fingers' or 'now tighten your shoulders' and we all feel the same thing - muscle tension! With a simple sequence of nine figures, everyone can get started with my Modern Tai Chi.

You then decide for yourself how to continue. You can stick to my short training sequence and enjoy the positive effects on your body and mind in an uncomplicated way. With my practical tips, the basic sequence gives rise to almost endless exercise options, which are always fun for everyone when modified. However, you can also supplement the sequence with elements of classic Tai Chi, for example.

To get you started, let's take a look at how today's Tai Chi has developed over the centuries from Asian teachings: what exactly is Tai Chi, what does it do and how can it help us to get to grips with ourselves again?

2.1 Background of Asian Tai Chi

Movement, meditation and therapeutic exercise have been popular in China for a long time. They developed from weaponless self-defence and were discovered as exercise systems with a high health value and have been continuously developed in more recent times.

In Beijing, for example, a Tai Chi form was compiled by the government in 1956 and given the name Beijing Form. A Tai Chi manual was sold in millions in China. This quickly became the basis of practice for young and old alike. As Tai Chi Chuan (in standard Chinese: Taijiquan) is usually practised before sunrise, it is also known as 'shadow boxing'. This is probably because the practitioners can only be recognised dimly in the twilight and it looks as if the Tai Chi practitioner is fighting against an imaginary opponent.

Tai Chi has thus evolved from a martial art and has taken on a new peaceful meaning today. It is an art of movement and health exercise on the one hand, and a meditation with a philosophical background on the other.

A Chinese proverb says: 'Those who practise Tai Chi regularly in the right way become as strong as a wood-cutter, as supple as a child and as calm as a sage'.

2.2 The art of movement of Asian Tai Chi

Tai Chi is like the endless flow of many successive waves. These draw their strength from the centre of the body, in Chinese 'Qi Hai' (an area three centimetres below the navel), and flow out into infinity. It is an endless sequence of ying and yang movements. A ying movement means that the body moves backwards and the arms move downwards and inwards, and a yang movement means that the body pushes forwards and the arms move upwards and outwards.

The slow, soft and flowing movements of Tai Chi lead to inner peace and balance, concentration and endurance in harmony with our natural breathing rhythm. Tai Chi prevents overexertion and injuries and is equally suitable for young and old, strong and weak, women and men. You don't need any special equipment and can practise every day and (almost) anywhere, regardless of the weather or time of year.

Do it! Regular practice allows you to feel the inner strength of your body again. It awakens your vitalising

Qi, which literally means energy, breath or also temperament and strength. Through regular Tai Chi exercises, your Qi can flow through your body again in a balanced way.

2.3 Basic movements and techniques

Tai Chi Chuan was long known as 'the boxing of the 13 forms' and consists of five basic movements and eight basic techniques:

The five basic movements are:

1. Procedure
2. Go back
3. Look to the left
4. Look to the right and
5. Centring your stable balance.

These basic movements are assigned to the Chinese elements wood, fire, earth, metal and water.

This results in the eight basic techniques:

6. Defence (Peng)
7. Reject (Lu)
8. Press (Chi)
9. Bumping (On)
10. Pulling (Tsai)
11. Disconnect (Lieh)
12. Elbow strike (Chou) and
13. Shoulder thrust (Kao).

These basic techniques represent the four cardinal points as well as south-west, north-east, north-west and south-east.

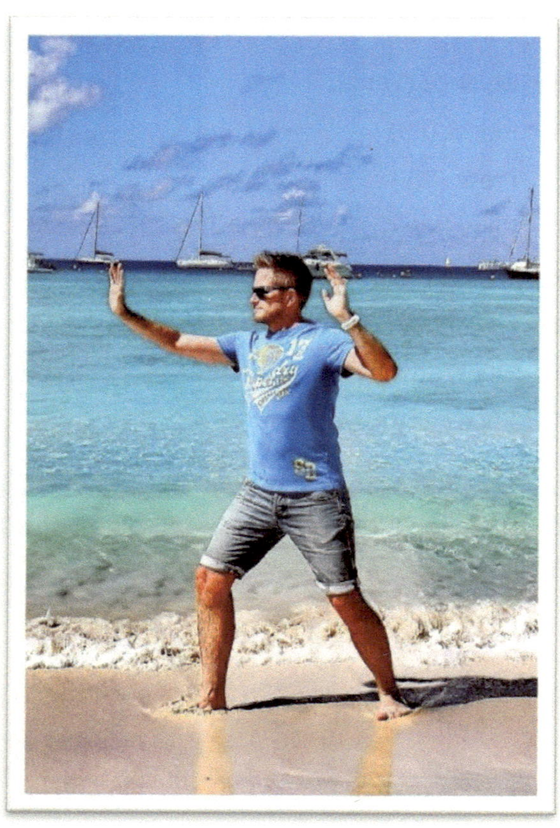

Simply practise anywhere in the world

3. Asian and Modern Tai Chi create a sense of well-being

In Tai Chi, we move our entire body in three-dimensional movements and do not spare any region. The aim is always to utilise as many parts of our organism as we can at the same time. This means that we will challenge and feel our entire organism more and more from the very beginning.

Let's take a look together at the positive effects that regular practice of our Tai Chi has on the various aspects of your body.

3.1 Effect on the nervous system

Tai Chi not only moves and strengthens the muscles and joints, but also the breathing. In particular, the 'up and down of the diaphragm' massages the organs in your abdomen, increases your breathing volume and has a calming effect on the central nervous system via the body's own receptors.

There is also scientific evidence that conscious breathing has positive effects on the body. Neurobiologists in Chicago (USA), for example, have established a direct link between conscious breathing and brain activity. Conscious breathing - such as nasal breathing - has been shown to change blood flow and activity in individual parts of the brain. This shows that our breathing influences our metabolism, brain activity and other body systems. Conscious and coordinated breathing in Tai Chi can also unfold its positive effects in this way.

Another decisive factor for the health-promoting effect of Tai Chi is the constantly straightened spine when practising. The posture resembles a marionette that is held by an invisible thread at the head. The vertebrae line up in a relaxed and natural way, like a string of pearls, until they are pulled towards the floor by a gently tilted pelvis. This posture and movement during practice straightens you out both internally and externally. This increases your ability to concentrate and brings about inner calm and balance. At the same time, mobility improves and innate reflexes are (re-)activated.

Thanks to the overall increase in blood flow and thus improved oxygen supply to our brain, insomnia, tiredness and states of agitation such as nervousness, emotional dissatisfaction, migraines and nervous weaknesses disappear or can be reduced without the use of medication.

3.2 Effect on the cardiovascular and pulmonary system

The belief that Tai Chi is only for relaxation and general well-being falls short of the mark. This would not be good either, because the lack of physical movement that our often sedentary way of working today often leads to muscle weaknesses. This has a detrimental effect on posture (e.g. hunched back, bow legs, spinal curvature, pelvic obliquity) as well as on blood circulation.

When it comes to postural problems, we often pay too much attention to the noticeably tense and painful muscles instead of recognising that these are the result of a muscle weakness that the body is trying to compensate for through poor posture. According to the rules of Chinese diagnostics, this means that a weakness in Ying (i.e. individual muscle groups) leads to an abundance of Yang (in this case tension).

Based on this idea, the 'healthy movement theory' ensures that imbalances in the muscles and posture are harmonised: hunched shoulders are loosened; a curved back is strengthened; knees that fall inwards are opened and the outer muscles of the legs are strengthened. The resulting 'feel-good tension' drives the blood in the veins and the life energy Qi in the meridians, supports the pumping activity of the heart and can therefore help with cardiac insufficiency, for example.

Regular breathing when practising Tai Chi increases the volume of your breath. Your breath becomes deeper as the diaphragm adapts better to the breathing movement. This allows blood to flow more easily to the lungs and back to the heart, which facilitates gas exchange. This allows larger quantities of oxygen to be exchanged for the waste product carbon dioxide from the body. The resulting improved oxygen supply to the entire body strengthens all your vital functions.

Many people breathe very superficially throughout their lives and only utilise a fifth of their breathing volume. This is usually because they only breathe with their mouth and upper chest. During deep breathing, the diaphragm, which is actively moved during Tai Chi, massages the abdominal organs, works down to the pelvic floor and up to the neck muscles via the shoulder girdle. The liver, which is connected to the diaphragm, is massaged the most, which prevents blood congestion in the liver. This term from Chinese medicine corresponds to the symptoms of right heart failure in Western medicine.

The more you move, the deeper you breathe. If you suffer from a lack of movement and breathing, the blood is poorly transported to the right side of the heart and from there to the lungs for gas exchange. Symptoms can then include heart failure with shortness of breath, oedema in the lungs, face and ankles, weak connective tissue with a predisposition to haemorrhoids and varicose veins, swelling of the liver and many more.

Chinese studies have shown that regular Tai Chi exercises strengthen the heart muscle, stabilise the cardio-vascular system, activate the metabolism and increase lung capacity, chest activity (in the case of ossification of the ribs and sternum cartilage) and lung ventilation.

Tai Chi thus effectively prevents chronic civilisation and age-related diseases!

3.3 Effect on posture

The postures in Asian Tai Chi have rather philosophical names: 'the wild horse shakes its mane', 'the monkey backs away', 'the crane lifts its wings'. It quickly becomes clear that many Tai Chi movements have emerged from the observation of animals. In fact, we can learn a great deal about natural forms of movement from animals.

Watch how young cats play: they stalk carefully and attentively, advancing slowly and quietly foot by foot, pausing and centring themselves before they - concentrating their strength - pounce on their opponent's playmate. The latter absorbs this onrushing force just as softly and lets itself roll away. Although a cat seems to mobilise '100 HP' through its vigilance, it does not tense up and retains its soft suppleness and centredness despite all its strength. It can even fall from a tree and still land safely back on its four paws while spinning.

As a result, natural movement patterns are an important aspect of strengthening our body in a comprehensive and balanced way. This insight forms the basis of Tai Chi, which aims to train the conscious experience of breathing, movement, posture and behaviour for our everyday lives.

During practice, you may notice unnatural tension caused by unaccustomed strain on individual untrained muscles. These are signs of muscular imbalances that can be corrected through regular Tai Chi. In this way, you can gradually find your way back to healthy muscular suppleness.

Our inner attitude is also visible in our outer attitude. Our way of thinking, acting and feeling is reflected in our outer appearance. Conversely, our inner personality develops through external impressions.

Tai Chi enables you to become aware of your breathing, your body and your movements through alert concentration. It is an ongoing process of discovery, the goal of which is a holistic harmony (thinking, feeling & acting) of your entire physical strength. In comparison, conventional gymnastics - such as squats, for example - is a mechanical strain that at best causes sweat and fatigue. In Tai Chi, on the other hand, the exercises refresh and relax you physically and mentally. These positive effects often carry over into your everyday activities, so that you become more aware of your own and other people's feelings and can deal with them better.

Tai chi also teaches you to master the unfamiliar, as both sides of the body and both sides of the brain are constantly exercised. The result is a physical, mental and emotional balance that is achieved through the combination of gymnastics and conscious body awareness.

3.4 Effect through the body position

In Tai Chi, the movements have a floating, dance-like effect and should be performed loosely and lightly, like clouds in the sky.

The correct Tai Chi posture gives you an optimal body position: the legs are neither too far apart nor too close together, the posture is shoulder-width apart. The spine is stretched both upwards and downwards. This is made easier by bending the knees slightly until the kneecap is above the forefoot. Now tilt your hips slightly forwards so that you feel a hollow back and do not tense your abdominal and lower back muscles. Your neck muscles are slightly stretched, as if you were hanging your spine upwards on a string like a marionette. This posture helps you to achieve correct and healthy spinal statics.

Many complaints in the neck, shoulder girdle, head and lumbar spine are the result of incorrect spinal statics caused by unnatural walking and standing. One advantage of correct posture is the distribution of the pressure wave during the breathing process. If the lumbar spine is curved too much, it protrudes too far into the abdominal cavity and pushes the organs forwards and downwards. However, the breathing movement can only be evenly distributed to the pelvic floor, the pelvic organs and the abdominal wall if the lumbar spine is as straight as possible. The Tai Chi posture releases the diaphragm so that breathing can connect the upper and lower half of the body. This results in deeper abdominal breathing.

In Tai Chi, we learn to breathe deeply and evenly again and to relax our diaphragm through conscious breathing. The breathing space increases and the expansion of the chest and abdomen creates 'new space for our joie de vivre'.

4. Modern Tai Chi translates Tai Chi into European

My Modern Tai Chi is a Europeanised form of this evolved Asian art of movement. It retains all of its aforementioned philosophical and physical origins, visualisations and possibilities.

As we Westerners are used to following structured, logical instructions, we find it difficult to understand the classic Asian image sequences and achieve the desired physical and mental effects. I therefore break down the classic sequences of images into structured, logical individual steps and present you with a form consisting of nine figures that covers all the important aspects of the exercise.

4.1 The logic bridge makes practising easier

For newcomers to Tai Chi, for example, the image of 'moving like a tree in the wind' is difficult to perform correctly, very late or often not at all. As a result, the desired physical effects do not materialise. Instructions such as 'spread your fingers', on the other hand, develop the same feeling of body tension in every practitioner and are easy to implement, as is the instruction 'one step forwards'.

Through this 'logic bridge', we Modern Tai Chi practitioners very quickly - often already in the first session - achieve the kind of body awareness that is desired in Asian Tai Chi and are motivated by this sense of achievement to continue working on our own Tai Chi. The Modern Tai Chi sequence can be practised for life but can also be switched to other Tai Chi styles or expanded to include other styles later on.

In addition to this European instruction, Modern Tai Chi also involves a special relationship between the participants and their instructor. In Asian Tai Chi, instruction is given by a master who sees himself as emotionally superior to his students and must be equally respected. As a participant in Asian Tai Chi, I am therefore always inferior to my teachers. In Modern Tai Chi, this bond is completely removed, and we adapt it to European training: We are all on the same level. Practitioners and instructors are on an equal footing, which is why the instructor is deliberately called the 'instructor'.

4.2 A quick sense of achievement

In the Modern Tai Chi courses I have been running since 2003, I have been surprised and very pleased to find that after practising the nine-figure sequence just once, every newcomer to the course has reported enthusiastically about the 'good body feeling' they have acquired. This sense of achievement has inspired many of them to continue working with and on themselves in exactly the same way.

In the next chapter I will first explain the general basic principles of practising Modern Tai Chi and in the following two chapters we will go through the individual exercise steps and the overall sequence one after the other.

Take advantage of my Europeanised form of Tai Chi now: try it out, feel inside yourself and look forward to quickly achieving your own success with the steps and exercises of my Modern Tai Chi, which I explain in detail.

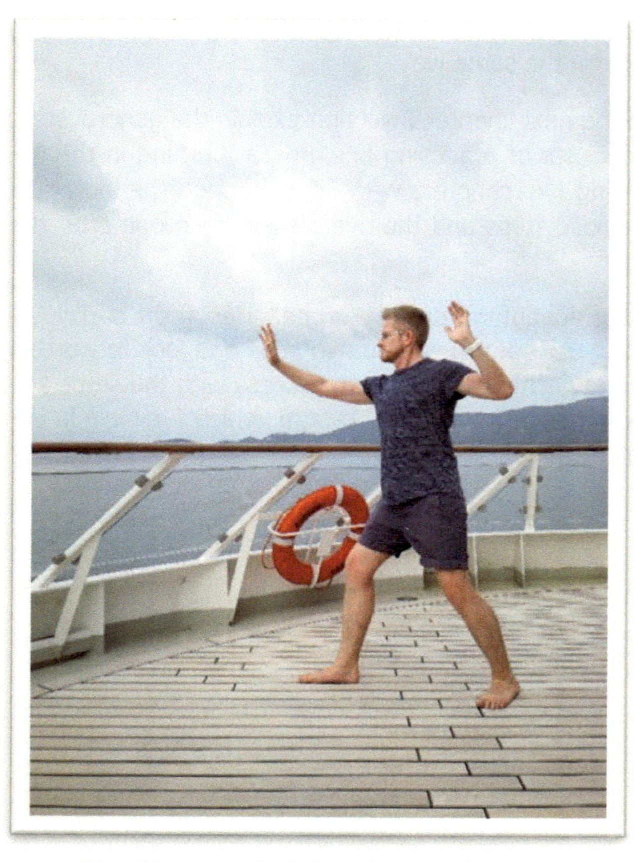

Stand in a comfortable place and practise

5. Modern Tai Chi practice tips

You don't need any special conditions or expensive equipment to practise Modern Tai Chi. You should simply wear comfortable clothes in which you feel good and can move freely.

I recommend a quiet room, balcony or garden as a place to start practising. However, you can also find a quiet place in a park, on the beach, by a lake or in the forest. The main thing is that you can practise there without any major disturbances.

If you like, a mirror can also be helpful from time to time so that you can look at yourself and control your movements. This way, you can deepen your body awareness and make corrections to your movements. However, be very honest with yourself and don't force anything.

5.1 Modern Tai Chi training

My Modern Tai Chi is a three-dimensional, whole-body form of movement that engages our entire organism with head, arms, torso and legs. If we look at it from the point of view of our European training theory, regular, effective and controlled Modern Tai Chi training has the following effects:

- Active muscle relaxation training

- Muscle stretching

- Training for concentration and (inner) balance

- Active body awareness training

- Active breathing training

- Build up physical resilience

- Stress reduction

- Active Qi training to maintain vitality and a positive attitude to life

- Combining movement and meditation for a balanced mental state

5.2 The eight basic principles

In all styles of Tai Chi, it is important that we do not act out the exercises like an actor, but endeavour to consciously experience them and continue to grow in them. This also applies to Modern Tai Chi. It therefore requires learning with conscious awareness of our movement!

For successful regular practice, please observe the following eight generally valid basic principles of Tai Chi:

1. **Still:** concentrate on your movement and breathing. Side thoughts should be switched off.

2. **Upright:** develop a feeling as if your head is being held by a golden cord. Your body follows your eyes and your eyes follow your consciousness.

3. **Relax:** try to be relaxed internally and externally to stimulate the flow of blood and breathing.

4. **Smooth:** the movements take place without interruption and flow smoothly into one another.

5. **Round:** your arms are round - like a ball without corners, protrusions or dents.

6. **Balanced:** do not overstretch large movements, do not shrink small movements.

7. **Stable:** always stand stable on both feet. It is a constant change between loose and firm.

8. **Sinking:** be stable and firm on the outside, flexible and supple on the inside, your

movements always take place around the centre of your body.

While practising, always focus your attention on just one of these eight principles. As a result, over time your body movement, breathing and mental awareness will merge into a meditative movement technique that has a healing effect on your entire organism.

5.3 The training goals

In addition to the eight principles, it also helps to con-sciously focus on one of the following training goals:

- a balanced overall well-being,
- relaxed muscles,
- stress reduction,
- reduce headaches, back pain or joint pain,
- a better perception of your own body,
- increases physical vigour,
- promoting a more relaxed daily routine,
- before exams or difficult appointments: pro-mote calmness and calm breathing and be able to concentrate on the essentials,

- in the evening: let go of everyday life and switch off, restful sleep.

5.4 Develop your Modern Tai Chi

Make sure that you feel comfortable in your movements. Seeing yourself in a positive light and feeling beautiful, graceful and powerful in your movements makes a huge contribution to your well-being. Try to consciously create these feelings in yourself when you practise. This has nothing to do with vanity. Rather, it is about giving our senses the opportunity to recognise more beauty and positivity. At the same time, this approach encourages you to perform the movements evenly and calmly. Notice your own charisma and enjoy it!

For the execution of the Modern Tai Chi movements, please keep the following points in mind:

- The forward stepping position is shoulder-width apart. Bend your knees slightly towards the tips of your toes so that the kneecap hovers over your forefoot and you can always see the tips of your toes.

- Always perform the individual steps first without shifting your weight. Only when your heel - or your entire foot when walking backwards - touches the ground, do you slowly shift your body weight onto this leg.
- When shifting your weight, always try to keep the centre of your body in the middle between your legs, and your body tension will give you a feeling of stability.
- Avoid any stretching. The suppleness in Modern Tai Chi movements is never achieved by stretching, but by utilising all the movement possibilities in the joint spaces. Always keep your joints slightly bent and never stretched!
- Avoid overstretching, even if it seems to make a movement easier at first - e.g. getting lower in the 'snake' figure. Trust your body, give it time to find its way into the movement sequences and develop in the process.
- Try to approach each repetition of the Modern Tai Chi form a little more relaxed than the

previous one. This will make your body feel cosy and pleasant all round.

6. Modern Tai Chi figures

In comparison to the variants already mentioned in Asian Tai Chi, such as the Beijing form with 24 figures or even more than 70 in some forms, we only deal with nine figures in Modern Tai Chi.

You can stay with these nine figures for the rest of your life. With the training principles outlined in the previous chapter, you can use them to create an almost endless range of training options, tackle new aspects each time and always have a good time.

When you start learning the Modern Tai Chi form, please breathe at all. Some people forget to breathe when they are concentrating on the movement and tension. First get into the flow of movement and feel your body as comfortable.

Once you're more familiar with it and your breathing is consistent, you can focus on the details of breathing: when should I breathe and for how long, and do I have to make my movements longer or shorter?

To help you, start by translating 'inhale' as 'in one direction' and 'exhale' as 'in the other direction'. This will help you to move more calmly and gradually become more confident in your Modern Tai Chi figure.

To help you start practising Modern Tai Chi, I will give you a time slot of 15 minutes. This is enough time for you to successfully concentrate on your movements, your muscle tension and your overall body awareness.

As a final tip, try the following figures one by one and feel their effect on your body. If you are confident with the figure and it feels good, then move on to the next figure and achieve the same level of comfort with it.

For each of the following nine exercises:

Practise these movements alternately to the right and left for as long as you want to practise.

6.1 Beginning

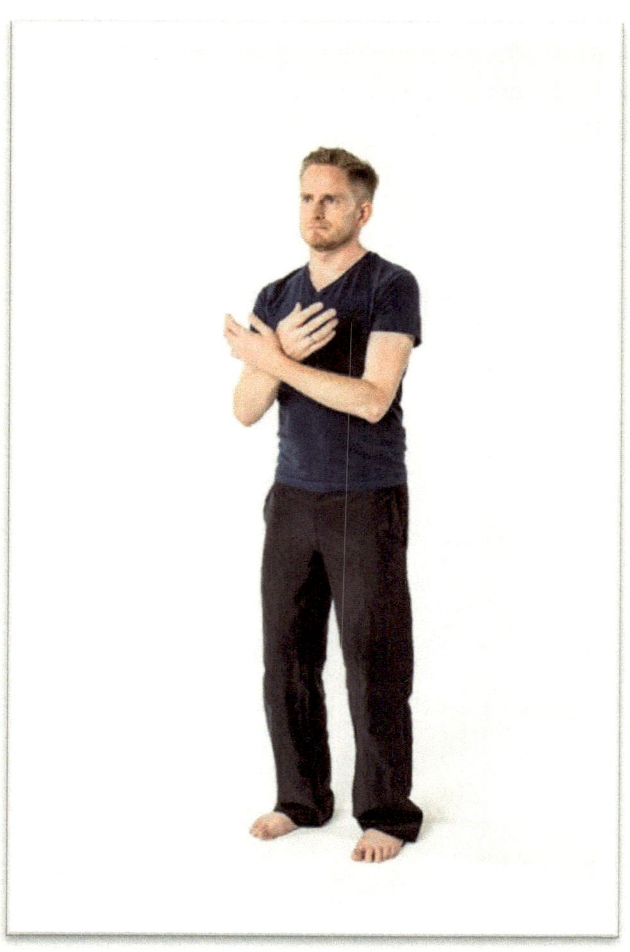

Short name: Beginning

Starting position: Stand with your feet shoulder-width apart. Your knees are slightly bent and you pull your feet and knees together towards the centre so that you feel the muscles on the inside of your thighs tense.

Your pelvis is only slightly tilted forwards, you pull your belly button inwards, keep your shoulders slightly pulled back and down and cross your wrists in front of your chest.

Movement execution:

To inhale, let both hands fall to the left and right of your pelvis with the backs of your hands first. At the same time, let the front of your pelvic crest drop down so that you come into a slight hollow back. As you do so, feel how the air you inhale comfortably fills your chest.

To exhale, first turn your palms round and lift them up to shoulder height with the backs of your hands in front of you, keeping them shoulder-width apart. To do this, lift your front iliac crest back up, tighten your gluteal muscles and pull your belly button inwards.

6.2 Rolling the little red ball

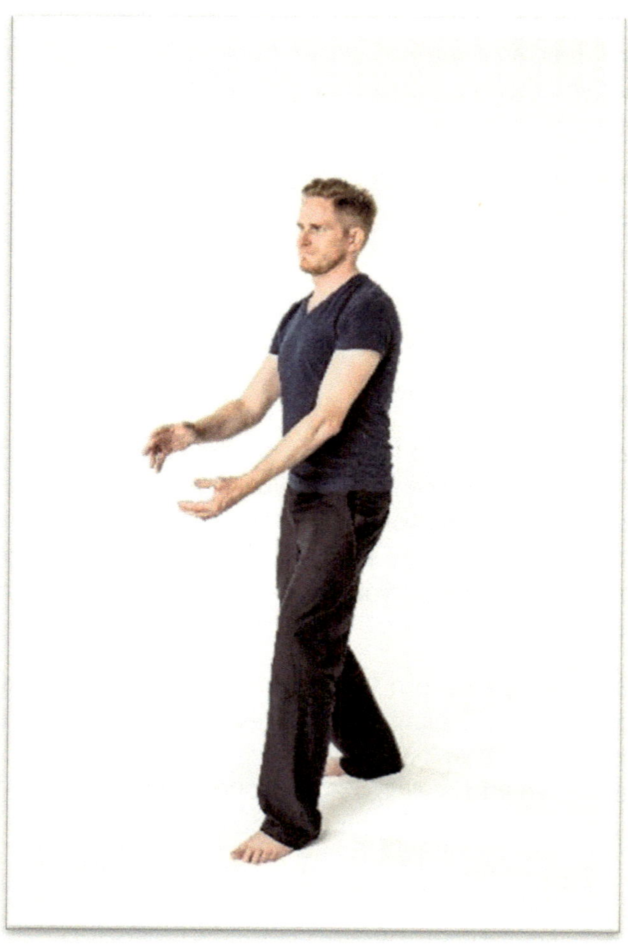

Short name: Defence

Starting position: Stand in a stride position with your feet shoulder-width apart and your stride length chosen so that it represents a small step forwards. Keep your knees bent, your pelvis slightly arched, your belly button pulled in and start with your weight on your back right leg. Keep your hands above your back foot at pelvic level as if you were holding a small red round ball.

Movement execution:

To exhale, first push your pelvis forwards so that you can still see your left toenails in front of your left knee-cap. At the same time, roll the small red round ball forwards and upwards over your left knee to shoulder height.

To inhale, pull your pelvis back again and roll the ball back down to the right of your pelvis. At the end points of this movement, keep turning the ball round in your hands.

6.3 Press your hands forwards

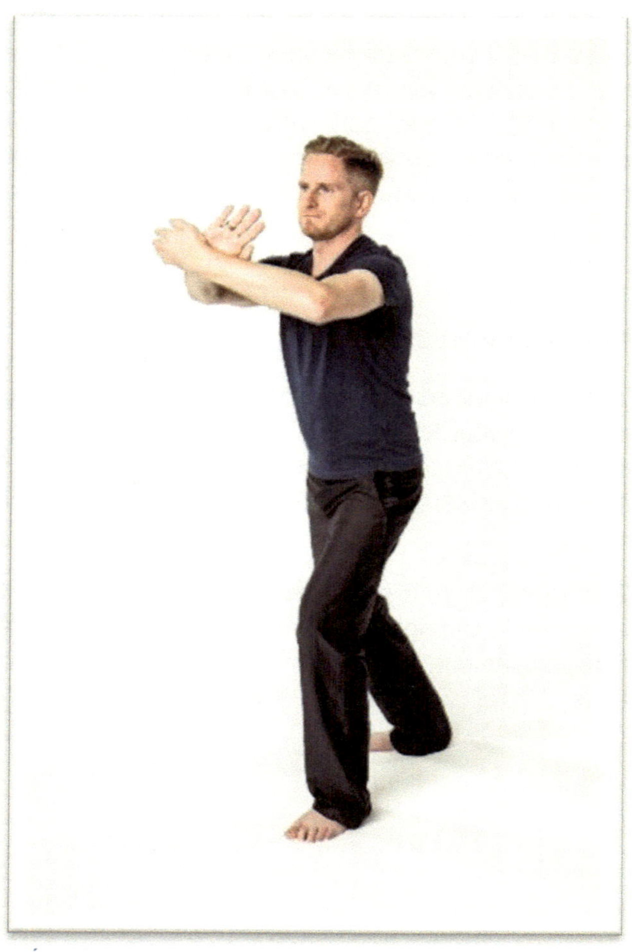

Short name: Presses

Starting position: Stand in a stride position with your feet shoulder-width apart and your stride length chosen so that it represents a small step forwards. Always keep your knees bent, your pelvis slightly arched, your belly button tucked in and start with your weight on your back right leg. Keep your hands above your back foot at pelvic level as if you were holding a small red round ball.

Movement execution:

To inhale, start to lift the small red round ball to the right of your body up to shoulder height.

To exhale, push your pelvis forward and your right hand presses your left forearm forward at shoulder height until your crossed hands are centred in front of your chest with your elbows bent.

To inhale, pull your pelvis back again and drop your hands down to the right of your pelvis and from there lift them back up to shoulder height to the right of your body.

6.4 Pull your elbows back to shoulder height

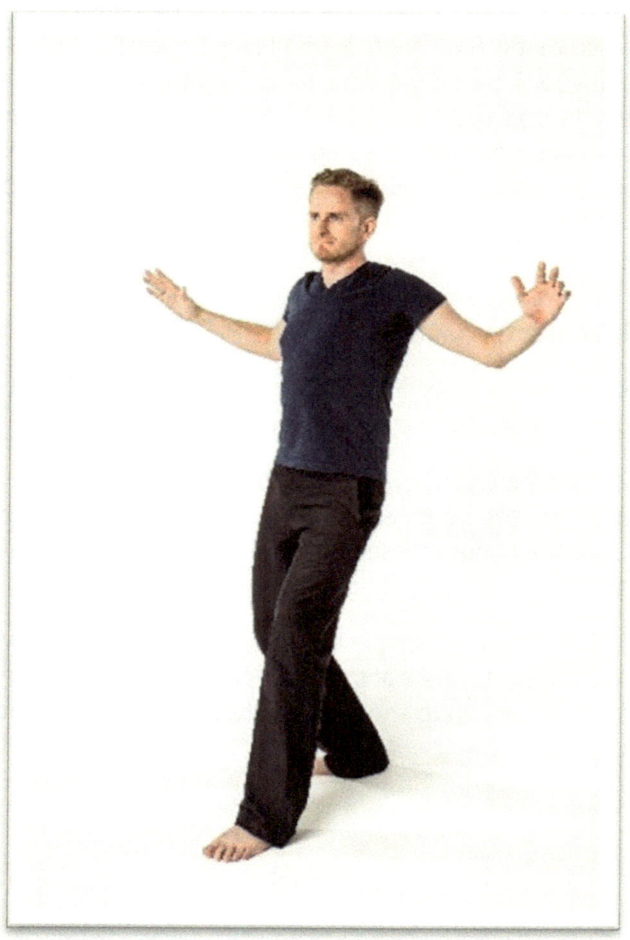

Short name: Pulling

Starting position: Stand in a stride position with your feet shoulder-width apart and your stride length chosen so that it represents a small step forwards. Keep your knees bent at all times, your pelvis slightly arched, your belly button pulled in and start with your weight over your front left leg. Your right wrist presses against the front of your left wrist. Both joints are centred in front of you at chest height with your elbows slightly bent.

Movement execution:

To inhale, first pull your pelvis back and your elbows directly back at shoulder height so that your shoulder blade muscles are pulled together strongly. Then drop your elbows down and feel the rotation of your shoulder blades clearly and pull your hands down with your elbows slightly bent so that your shoulders are pulled down just as strongly.

To exhale, first push your pelvis forwards again and then push your palms and arms forwards with your elbows slightly bent and cross your wrists in front of your chest, looking into the centre of your palms.

6.5 Push your hands forwards

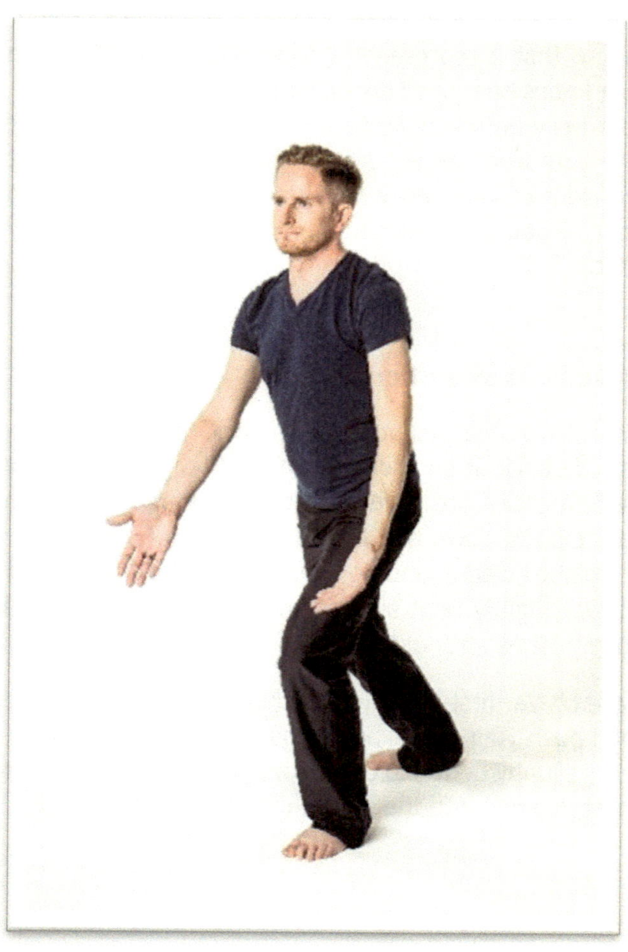

Short name: Jolting

Starting position: Stand in a stride position with your feet shoulder-width apart and your stride length set so that it represents a small step forwards. Keep your knees bent at all times, your pelvis slightly arched, your belly button pulled in and start with your weight over your front leg. To do this, press your right wrist forwards against your left wrist and, with your elbows slightly bent, look into the centre of your palms at chest height in front of you.

Movement execution:

To inhale, move your pelvis back and pull your palms down so that both hands are level with your pelvis. Then pull your shoulder blades together strongly and straighten up.

To exhale, push your pelvis forward again and use the muscle tension built up between your shoulder blades to push your palms forwards again, turning them so that you can look back in until you press your wrists together in the centre of your chest.

6.6 Whip lash

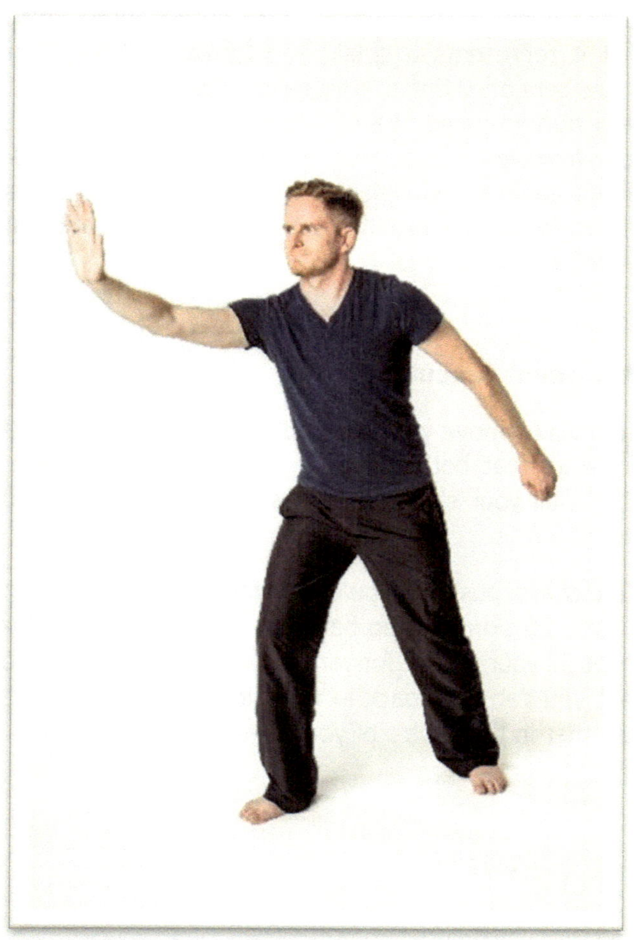

Short name: Whip

Starting position: Stand in a walking stance with your feet shoulder-width apart. Start with your weight on your back right leg, press your wrists against each other and look into the centre of your palms at chest height in front of you.

Movement execution:

To inhale, first shift your weight forwards and pull your hands closer to your chest. Finally, stand on your left leg, move your crossed wrists to the left towards your shoulder and lift your back leg off the floor.

To exhale, place the heel of your right foot turned ninety degrees outwards and shift your weight back onto your right leg. To do this, move your right elbow forwards to the right and finish with a whip with your right hand in a sweeping circular motion.

To inhale, shift your weight again, turn back and come to a standstill on your left leg. To do this, bring your hands towards each other again.

To exhale, bring your right foot back, put weight on your right leg and cross your wrists at chest height.

6.7 Snake

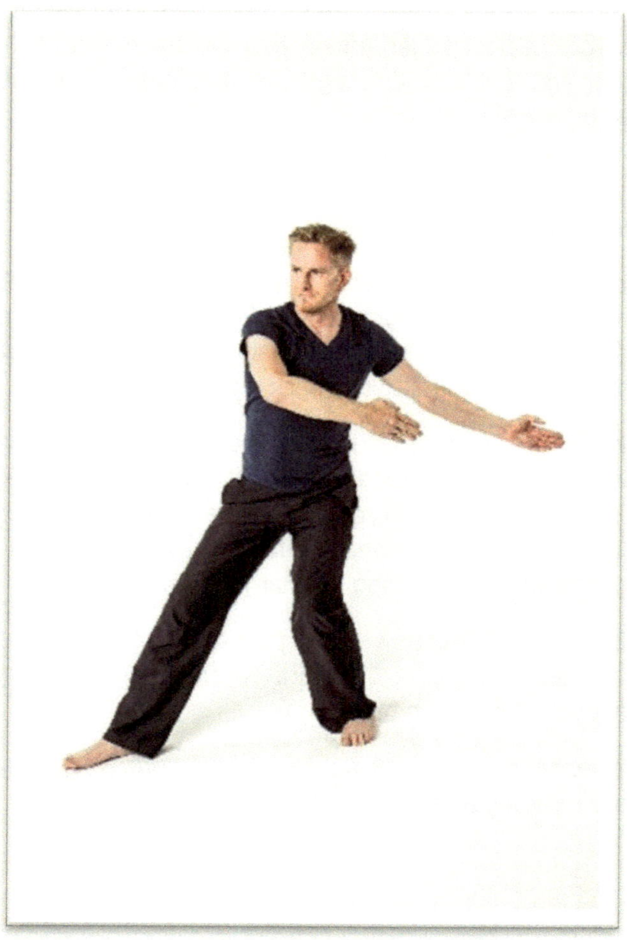

Short name: Snake

Starting position: Stand in a stride position with your feet shoulder-width apart and your stride length chosen to represent a small step. You start with your weight on your front right leg, holding your left hand behind you at shoulder height and your right palm facing forwards with a whip.

Movement execution:

To inhale, pull your hands together as if to grasp a small round red ball while pulling your weight onto your left leg. Now drop the imaginary ball, arch your spine intensely, roll the ball forwards at an angle, shift your weight onto your front right leg and turn your right foot outwards by around 45 degrees. To do this, slowly straighten up vertebra by vertebra until the ball reaches shoulder height.

To exhale, pull your weight back onto your left leg, go back with your left hand and open your hands with your shoulder blades together. Then push your weight forwards again and finish with a whip with your right hand so that your palm is pointing forwards.

6.8 Pheasant

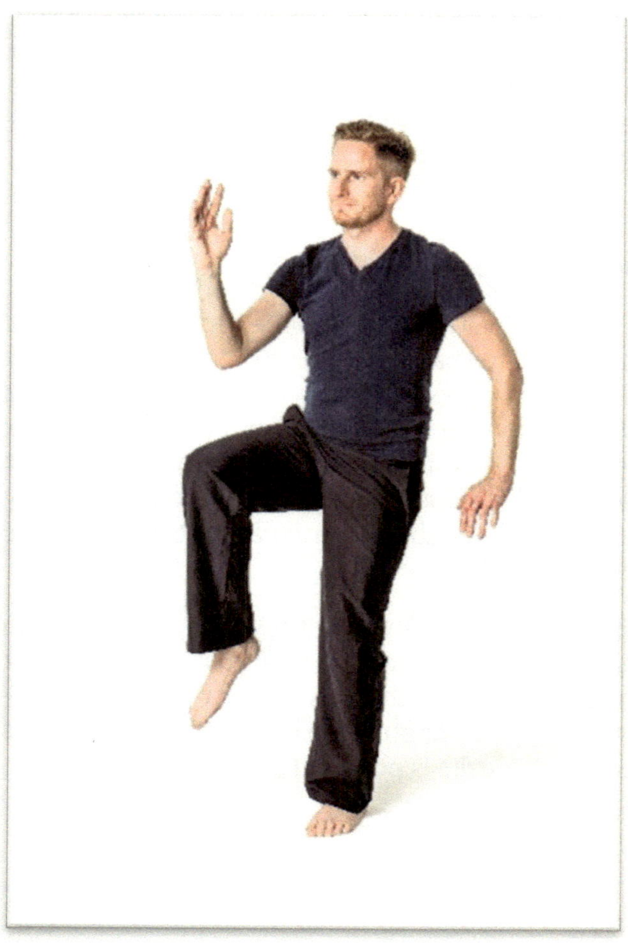

Short name: Pheasant

Starting position: Stand stable on your right foot and support your right hand to the right of your pelvis as if on an imaginary post. Keep your left leg lifted and point your toes towards the floor, while your left arm is raised above your lifted leg so that your left thumb is pointing towards your nose.

Movement execution:

To inhale, let your raised leg take a small step back and put equal weight on both legs. As you do this, first drop your raised arm down and then raise both hands back up to shoulder height. Your left hand is to the left of your body and your right forearm is horizontal in front of your torso.

To exhale, press your left hand down next to your pelvis to support yourself, keep your elbow slightly bent and at the same time lift your right leg up and point your toes towards the floor. Only when you have a stable stance on the left do you turn your right elbow downwards so that your right hand comes to the right of your head and your right thumb points towards your nose.

6.9 Monkey

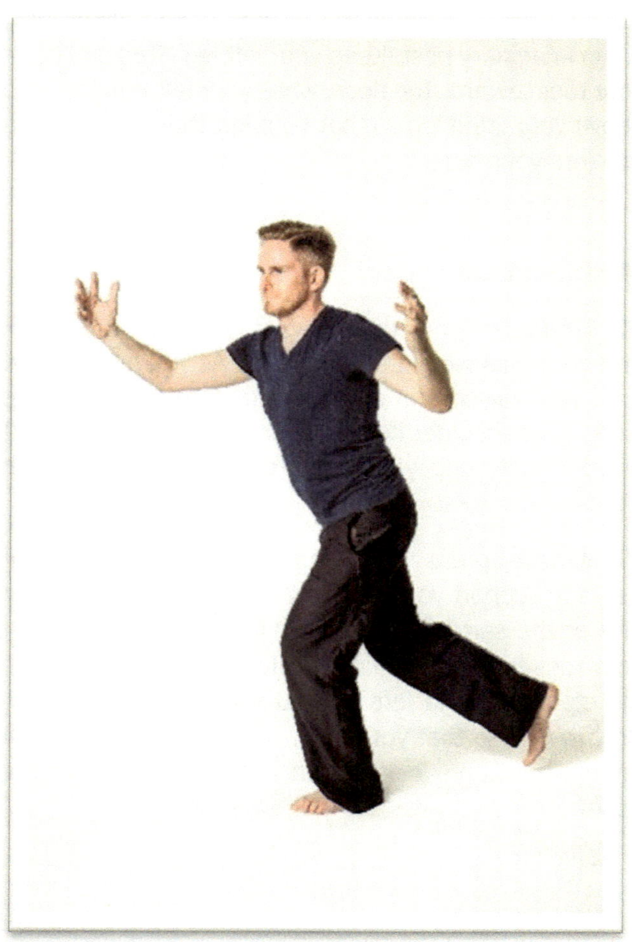

Short name: Monkey

Starting position: Stand stable on your right foot and support your right hand to the right of your pelvis as if on an imaginary post. Keep your left leg lifted and point your toes towards the floor, while your left arm is raised above your lifted leg so that your left thumb is pointing towards your nose.

Movement execution:

To inhale, open your arms to shoulder height. Raise your right hand to shoulder height while pulling your shoulder blades together. To do this, slowly bring your left foot back and only put it down with the tips of your toes when you feel tension in your left gluteal muscle.

To exhale, put all the weight on your left foot and pull your pelvis backwards. To do this, push your right hand forwards with your palm and pull your left palm to the left of your pelvis so that you can look into it and stand in a stable position.

6.10 Conclusion

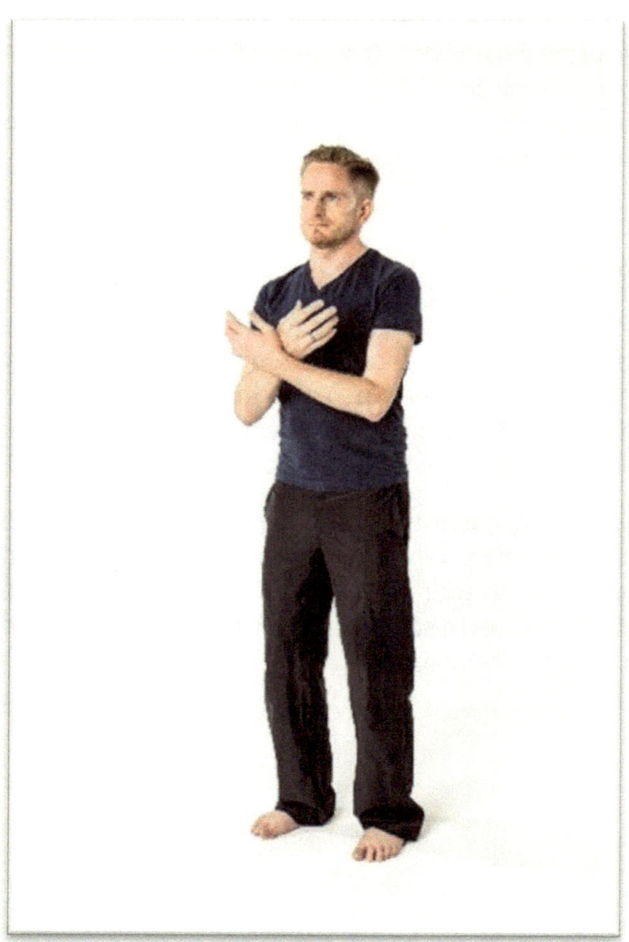

Short name: Degree

Final position: Stand with your feet shoulder-width apart. Your knees are slightly bent and you pull your feet and knees together towards the centre so that you feel the muscles on the inside of your thighs tense.

Your pelvis is only slightly tilted forwards, you pull your belly button inwards, keep your shoulders slightly pulled back and down and cross your wrists in front of your chest.

Movement execution:

As you inhale and exhale, enjoy the muscle tension you have built up in all your muscles. You can feel how it supports you, keeps your joints bent and you are up-right and can look forwards to breathe in a completely relaxed way!

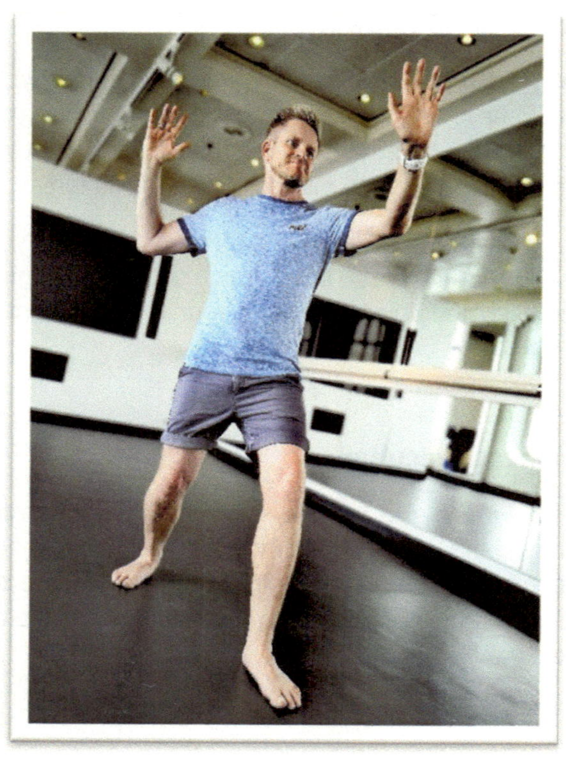

Just practise for 15 minutes every day

7. Modern Tai Chi Form

Having looked at these nine Modern Tai Chi figures individually, we now come to what we want to achieve in Tai Chi - my Modern Tai Chi form. In doing so, we put the figures we have just practised together and very quickly get into the pleasant flow of three-dimensional movements in our body.

Start with pieces one and two. Once you are confident with this, add the next piece at the end and so on. It is therefore not necessary to attach all nine pieces together straight away.

When you start learning the Modern Tai Chi form, please breathe at all. First get into the flow of movement and feel your body as comfortable.

Once you are more familiar with this and your breathing is consistent during your practice, you can focus on the details of breathing: when should I breathe and for how long, and do I have to make my movements longer or shorter?

To help you, translate 'inhale' as 'in one direction' and 'exhale' as 'in the other direction'. This will help you to move more calmly and gradually become more confident in your Modern Tai Chi form.

Form as a sequence of images

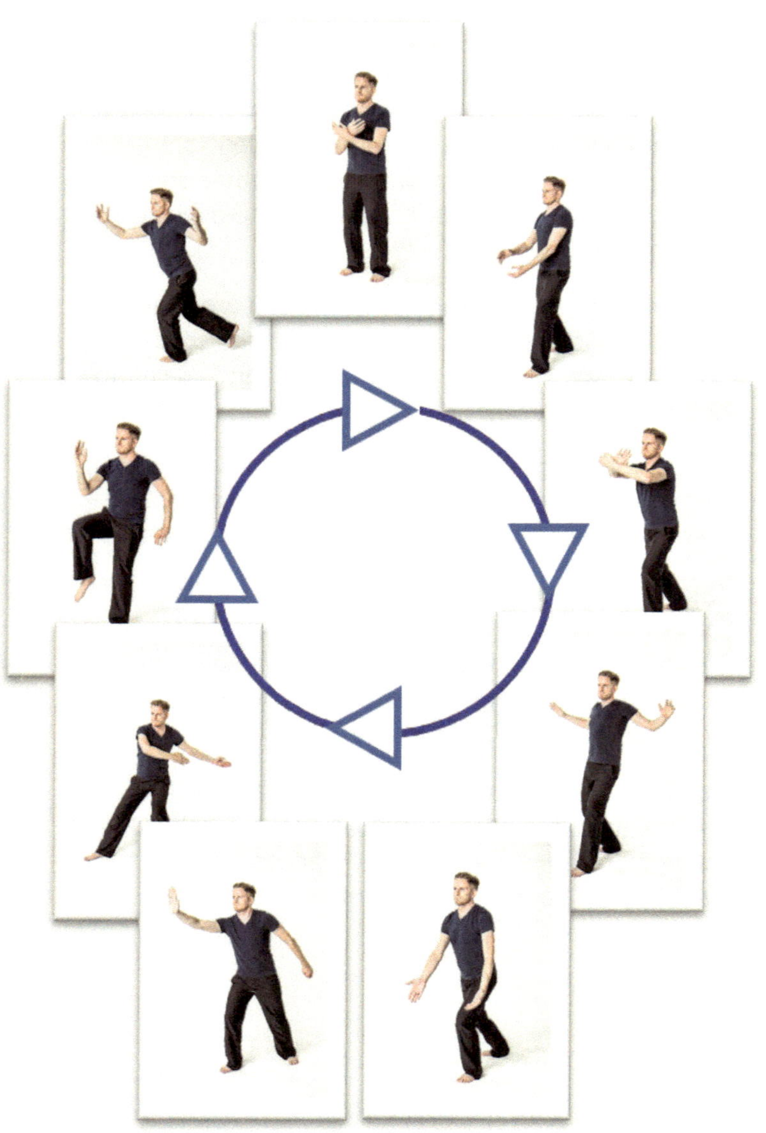

7.1 Explanations of the picture sequence

As with practising the individual Modern Tai Chi figures, we start with the Modern Tai Chi form with the 'beginning' figure, which you can see in the top centre of the left-hand diagram. From there we move clockwise to the bottom right and further to the left and top until we come back to the 'beginning'.

You can practise this sequence for as long as you feel comfortable. I advise you to take a break after four or six complete rounds, loosen up your muscles, shake them out and breathe in and out deeply. As a guide for your daily practice, I recommend at least 15 minutes. You are welcome to practise for longer, but for a good training effect you should not go below 15 minutes.

Here is a suggestion on how I teach my Modern Tai Chi in a class. It is normal for you to have difficulties coordinating your breathing and movement at the beginning. Please don't put yourself under pressure but accept that you will need time and practice to harmonise your breathing and movement. The important thing is to start by breathing at all during the exercises. As you gradually become more confident in the figures, your breathing and movement will also harmonise.

My Modern Tai Chi form for a beginner course:

Stand with both feet shoulder-width apart, keep your knees bent, pull your feet and knees towards the centre and feel the muscles in the middle of your thighs as tense and stabilising. To do this, tilt your pelvis slightly forwards, draw in your belly button and look at your palms crossed in the centre of your chest. Stand upright and stable, keeping your shoulders pulled back and down.

Start *inhaling* with a small step to the right, shift your weight evenly onto both legs and let your hands fall to the right and left of your pelvis.

To exhale, raise your hands back up to shoulder height, pull your iliac crest up and your belly button in.

To inhale, shift your weight onto your right leg and bring your hands together over your right thigh.

To exhale, remain as stable as possible up to your navel and move your hands in a large circular motion to the left and upwards until you grasp an imaginary small red round ball at 'one o'clock'.

To inhale, drop the ball to the right of your pelvis, lift your left heel slightly off the floor and come to a stop on your right leg.

To exhale, place your left heel on the floor with a small step forwards, keep your knees bent and continue to feel the muscle tension between the tips of your toes and your belly button. To do this, roll the small red round ball up until it reaches shoulder height above your left knee.

To inhale, pull your pelvis back again, keep the tension in your legs up to your belly button, roll the ball down to the right of your pelvis and lift it up from there to your right shoulder height.

To exhale, push your pelvis forwards again and maintain the muscle tension between your toes and belly button. To do this, your right hand pushes your left wrist forwards until it is centred at shoulder height and your elbows remain slightly bent.

To inhale, pull your pelvis back again with the tension between your toes and belly button. To do this, bring your elbows back to shoulder height until your shoulder blades are as close together as possible. Only then do you let your elbows drop and feel the rotation of your shoulder blades and your straightening and let your hands fall to the right and left of your pelvis.

To exhale, push your pelvis forwards again and maintain the tension in your muscles in your legs and pelvis. Now point your palms forwards, push them forwards with your elbows slightly bent and lift them until your hands are pressed together in the centre at chest height, revealing your palms.

To inhale, release your right heel and pull your pelvis forwards so that you come to a standstill on your left leg. Pull your clenched palms towards your chest, move them from there to your left shoulder and feel your pelvis rotate to the right.

To exhale, place your right heel 90 degrees apart and shift your weight onto both feet. Your left hand remains to the left of your body, while your right arm performs a large circular movement, elbow first, with a final whip stroke forwards.

To inhale, pull your pelvis back while your left hand and right hand slide towards each other and grab the small red round ball again halfway through. Drop it as low as possible and arch your spine. Now move the weight forwards again and roll the ball upwards so that it reaches shoulder height. Hold your left forearm horizontally in front of your chest and your right hand continues to hold the ball.

To exhale, pull your right hand up onto your right leg and support yourself with the palm of your hand next to your pelvis as if on a post. When you are stable on your right leg, lift your left knee up and turn your left elbow down so that your left thumb is pointing towards the tip of your nose.

To inhale, drop your left arm like your left leg, take a small step backwards and place your left foot firmly on the floor. To do this, raise your right arm up to shoulder height so that your right forearm is horizontal in front of your chest and raise your left hand back up to shoulder height to the left.

To exhale, pull your left hand up onto your left leg until the palm of your hand is resting on an imaginary post at pelvic level. When you are stable on your left leg, lift your right knee up and turn your right elbow downwards so that your right thumb is pointing towards the tip of your nose.

To inhale, first pull your shoulder blades together strongly and keep the tension in your hands and arms. Now push your right foot backwards and keep it in the air until you feel tension in your right gluteal muscle.

To exhale, place the toe of your right foot on the floor and shift your weight back onto both legs. Keeping the tension in your arms, push your left hand forward with the palm of your hand until it comes to rest at shoulder height with your elbow slightly bent. Pull your right hand down to the right of your pelvis so that you can spit into the palm of your hand.

To inhale, first pull your shoulder blades together strongly, lift your right hand up and turn your left hand so that both palms are facing each other. Now lift your left leg up and take a long, slow step backwards with it until you feel tension in your left gluteal muscle.

To exhale, place your left foot on the floor and shift your weight back onto both legs. Keeping tension in your arms, push your right hand and palm forwards until it comes to rest at shoulder height with your elbow slightly bent. Pull your left hand down to the left of your pelvis so that you can spit into the palm of your hand.

To inhale, turn your body to the left and let your left arm slide backwards in a large circular motion until your hands are at shoulder height on both sides. You also turn your right foot to the left and now feel upright and refreshed.

To exhale, pull your left foot shoulder-width apart towards your right, drop both hands in a large circular motion and lift them back up to the centre of your chest, crossing them over each other.

This form of movement is quite easy to learn with the 'turn to the right', as we humans are predominantly right-handed. Nevertheless, it is also important to learn the 'turn to the left'. However, the first time you turn to the left will feel very strange, as if you haven't practised Modern Tai Chi before. But don't worry, this feeling will disappear relatively quickly.

As a further increase after the first step of turning only to the right and then in the second step only to the left, in the third step you can perform a continuous alternating turn to the right and left. This allows you to challenge and strain your body in a targeted manner and thus compensate for one-sided movements in your everyday life, job or sport, for example.

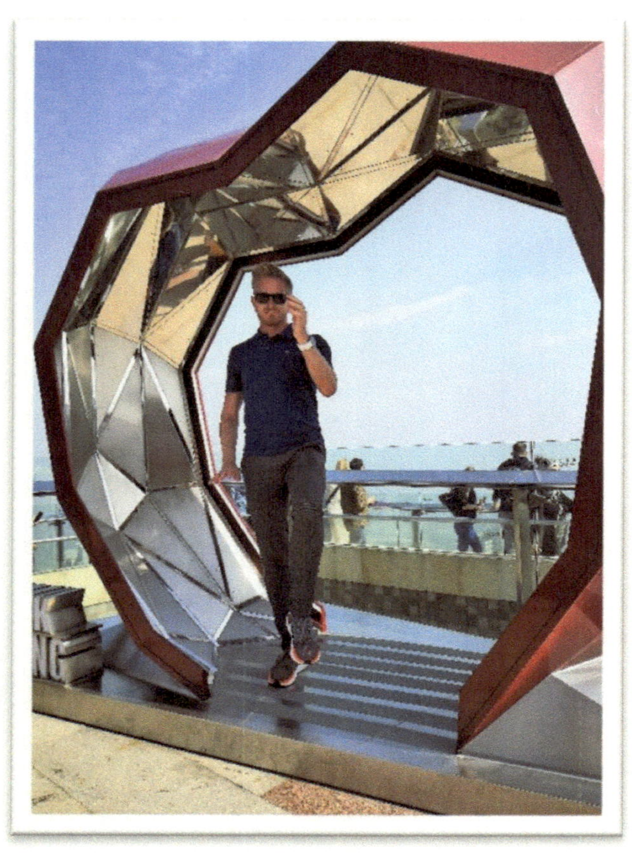

Develop your Modern Tai Chi

8. Develop Modern Tai Chi for yourself

If you have come this far, tried Modern Tai Chi and enjoyed this three-dimensional movement, then I am delighted to have taken you on this journey and hopefully you will enjoy your pleasant whole-body feeling during and after each practice!

What can you do now with what you have learnt here, where can and should you go?

The first thing I would like to say to you is that it is not important to keep looking forwards and creating more and more figures, more twists, more runs or whatever you are thinking about. This misdirected ambition would do more harm than good to the balancing effect of Modern Tai Chi. What is important to me personally as a trainer and practitioner of Modern Tai Chi is to become more and more confident with what I am doing right now and to be able to reproduce this stable and happy feeling easily and anywhere in the world at any time.

That doesn't sound like us Europeans, I agree. Our western culture is very one-sidedly focussed on the idea of performance. From my own experience as a high-performance swimmer, as a coach and as a doctor of sports medicine, training in a European way means developing as quickly as possible in the direction of 'higher, further and faster'. However, this also means that a lot of things fall by the wayside half-heartedly, even though they will later be needed as a secure basis for expansion and progress or will be absolutely necessary.

Here I would like to come back to the philosophies contained in Asian Tai Chi. Here, the focus is on careful and in-depth execution, the deeper and deeper engagement with one's own body based on the exercises learnt, the balancing of tension and relaxation, the even flow of breathing, concentration and energy throughout the entire organism. Your Modern Tai Chi should also focus on this.

So let's move forward as confidently and motivated as possible, and let's coordinate the content, time and place of our Modern Tai Chi practice accordingly. That way, we'll make successful progress together and feel good all round every time!

Time and technology make it possible for me to be at your side the way you want me to be. No matter where you live, where you travel and where you practice, I can be with you: via the internet, in my practice, on event trips or also with individually booked activities for you privately, at work or whatever we both think of.

On my website at **www.moderntaichi.training** you will always find everything up to date about me, what I offer and when and where I will be offering and realising something. Take a look around and let me know what else you're interested in.

Under '**modern tai chi training**' on the website I offer you information, video workouts, online courses, live courses as well as workshops, event trips or simply personal training with me to get ahead in the matter.

To make it easier for you to practise your Modern Tai Chi personally, I also have an exercise video on offer so that you always have me in front of you, can follow the exercises well and will therefore always be more stable and confident. Take a look online or contact me by email, WhatsApp or SMS and I will help you further.

With this in mind, I hope you continue to enjoy practising and developing your Modern Tai Chi and will always be happy to help you if you need help or motivation!

GR codes to more information, courses, travel, videos & my author page

WEB Modern Tai Chi

Author Tobias Block

9. References

p. 17: for the history of the Peking form, see e.g.: https://de.wikipedia.org/wiki/Taijiquan#Form, retrieved on 11/11/2021.

p. 21-22: on the connection between conscious nasal breathing and brain activity, see e.g: Zelano, Christina et. al: Nasal Respiration Entrains Human Limbic Oscillations and Modulates Cognitive Function. Journal of Neuroscience 7 December 2016, 36 (49) 12448-12467.

p. 25: For studies on the effects of Tai Chi exercise, see e.g: Yang G-Y, Wang L-Q, Ren J, Zhang Y, Li M-L, Zhu Y-T, et al. (2015) Evidence Base of Clinical Studies on Tai Chi: A Bibliometric Analysis. PLoS ONE 10(3): e0120655.

Picture credits

The rights to all images are held by Tobias Block.

Disclaimer

The advice and exercises in this book are aimed at physically and mentally healthy people. Anyone undergoing medical treatment or who feels ill should always speak to their doctor before starting to practise Modern Tai Chi.

The exercises, thoughts, methods and suggestions represent the opinion and experience of the author. They have been compiled by the author to the best of his knowledge and checked with the utmost care. However, they are no substitute for personal, competent medical advice. Each reader remains responsible for his/her own actions. The author can therefore accept no liability for any damage resulting from the practical exercises and advice given in the book or any printing errors.

The name **MODERN TAI CHI by tobias block** is a registered trade mark of Tobias Block. The material contained in this book and the exercise concept presented may not be reproduced, transferred or processed in any form without the written consent of the author.